Succeed at Living Gluten Free

By Pam Jordan

I'm a Celiac, LLC

ImaCeliac.com
@ImaCeliac

Succeed at Living Gluten Free

Succeed at Living Gluten Free

65 tips to help you

By Pam Jordan

ISBN- 13: 978-1497515604
ISBN -10: 1497515602

Self Published through Creative Space.

Editors: Nikki Smalling, Lindsay Dickerson, Mary
Tomczak, Cynthia Brewer, Rhonda Duell, Kelly
Malzewski, Erica Morales, Christina McGlynn,
Jennifer Spector, Francine Waltman,

Cover Design: Black Train Designs

Foreword

"Not only is Pam Jordan an amazing advocate for the Gluten Free world, she's witty, smart and makes delicious recipes. Pam has been through it all, just like you're experiencing now. Her book will shortcut you past all the little "whoops...now I knows" before you make the mistake yourself. She is the shoulder to lean on, to learn from, and to laugh with. You'll be glad you bought this book, now start reading."

Andrea Harper – Red Apple Lipstick
www.redapplelipstick.com

"When it comes to living Gluten Free, Pam Jordan knows all about that! Pam has been living the Gluten Free life since her Celiac Disease diagnosis. Pam has quickly become a well-known blogger and expert in the Gluten Free Community. Whether you are new to living Gluten Free or a seasoned veteran, this book is stocked with tips on how to survive when living Gluten Free. If you are looking to be successful in the world of 'Gluten Free', this survival guide which is packed with 65 simple Gluten Free Living Tips is a must have!"

Cindy Gordon – Vegetarian Mamma
www.vegetarianmamma.com

Acknowledgments

Thank you to the Gluten Free community for your continued support! I would not be here without you! Thank you to the many Gluten Free bloggers who I am blessed to call friends.

Thank you to my family who stands beside me for all my Gluten Free chaos. Thank you for eating my food and letting me take pictures of it.

A special thank you to my husband, Nick. I am better because of you! I love you!

Disclaimer

I am not a doctor, nor am I authorized to give medical advice. The information contained in this book comes from my personal opinion, thoughts and experiences. If you feel you have health issues, you should consult a medical professional.

Table of Contents

Succeed at Living Gluten Free

Introduction

What is Gluten?

Gluten is a protein found in wheat, flour, rye and barley. For people with Celiac Disease, Gluten sensitivity or a wheat allergy, digesting it can make them sick. Gluten affects everyone differently; some people get headaches, digestive issues, fatigue, bloating, and more.

Why go Gluten Free?

People start a Gluten Free lifestyle for different reasons. From my experience, there is normally a health related issue that causes someone to go Gluten Free. The top three reasons are Celiac Disease, Gluten sensitivity and a wheat allergy. I am Gluten Free due to a Celiac Disease diagnosis, in which the only treatment is a Gluten Free lifestyle. Whatever the reason, if you feel better without Gluten then live Gluten Free!

Why tips to help?

Living a Gluten Free lifestyle isn't easy. It is hard to know what is and what isn't safe. There are a ton of little things that you need to know to successfully live Gluten Free.

This easy to read guide will fill you with loads of information. Whether you are Gluten Free or a caregiver for someone who is Gluten Free these tips will help.

Whether you are a beginner or an old pro, you are bound to find a tip in here that will help you on your Gluten Free journey. Good luck and let me know if I can help!

Basic Gluten Free Eating

1. Eating Gluten Free is hard. It takes time and practice.

Congratulations on deciding to live a Gluten Free lifestyle, whether it was 5 days ago or 5 years ago. I don't want to burst your bubble but it is hard to live Gluten Free. There are many changes that will need to be made and you will need to approach food differently. Fear not, you can do this! This book has some great tips to help you along your journey. If you slip up or make a bad food choice, don't beat yourself up about it. Learn from the experience and move on. Even after years of being Gluten Free you can still make a mistake. Just keep trying, focus on living 100% Gluten Free and the good its doing for your body.

2. Gluten affects all of us differently.

Everyone reacts differently to Gluten and all our bodies have different combinations of problems due to it. The list of effects is large so I will just highlight a few here:

- Fatigue
- Headaches
- Bloating
- Constipation
- Diarrhea
- Weight gain
- Weight loss
- Skin rashes
- Depression
- Anxiety
- Infertility

3. Commit to a 100% Gluten Free lifestyle. Cheating is not an option.

Being Gluten Free is an all or nothing commitment. You need to let your body heal from ingesting Gluten for years. Living Gluten Free isn't about eating Gluten Free when it is convenient or easy, because if it were none of us would be Gluten Free. Living Gluten Free is about a lifestyle change that includes consuming only products without Gluten. Taking a bite of your favorite pizza isn't worth how sick it will make you feel.

4. Be prepared to learn how to read the labels on food.

You will need to be an expert food label reader. You will be able to scan a list of ingredients and know if it is safe to eat or not. Gluten hides in strange places and doesn't always stand out. With practice you will be able to spot Gluten among the strange names in food labels. Try not to eat any packaged food without first reading the label.

5. Be prepared to accidently feed yourself Gluten because you didn't read a label correctly.

The last tip talks about reading labels and you will get very good at this with practice. But know that ingredients change and you will have to be diligent even with food items you have used for years. I had a seasoning mix change ingredients and the new combination had wheat in it! Unfortunately I grabbed the box like normal and prepared a meal with it because I thought it was safe. Always read the label!

6. When in doubt, just don't eat it.

If you aren't sure if something is Gluten Free, just don't eat it. If the label is unclear or you can't ask the preparer questions, it is safest to simply avoid it. I have seen Gluten in items like canned beans, so don't just assume a food item is safe. When eating at a social gathering don't be afraid to ask questions and if safe options are not available, just don't eat.

7. Both wine and most distilled alcohol is Gluten Free.

The good news is both wine and distilled alcohol are Gluten Free. There are also a number of Gluten Free beers available. You will need to avoid malt beverages like wine coolers, hard lemonades and malt liquor. The labeling on alcohol is different than food, so you will need to check the product's website for a full listing of ingredients. You will also need to be cautious around flavored alcohols, as wheat is cheap filler and a flavor additive.

8. When you accidentally eat Gluten it is called being "Glutened".

The term for unintentionally ingesting Gluten is called being "Glutened". An example sentence is, "I feel horrible this morning! I must have been Glutened at the restaurant last night." This is a term commonly understood and used in the Gluten Free community. The timeline for knowing you have been Glutened depends on the amount of Gluten ingested and how your body reacts. Some people know right away, some an hour later, and some the next morning. If you have been Glutened it is important to trace your steps and figure out where it came from so you can avoid whatever caused you to be sick.

9. Wash your hands before you eat anything.

Never eat anything without first washing your hands. It is too hard to keep track of what you touched last to know if your hands are safe. If you live in a mixed Gluten Free home this is especially important. Even the refrigerator door handle can have Gluten hiding on it! Remember Gluten is sticky and likes to stick to surfaces, so it needs to be thoroughly washed off your hands. If soup and water are not available use alcohol based hand cleaners.

10. You will go through a mourning stage with the loss of Gluten in your life.

When you give up Gluten there are a lot of emotions that go along with this life change. You will experience food completely differently now. Going out for dinner with friends, holiday gatherings and business lunches will be different now. If you choose to be Gluten Free for the rest of your life, Gluten has essentially died to you. You may go through the stages of grief and loss. Many a tear has been shed after going Gluten Free. Know that it may be hard, know you are not alone and know you will survive.

11. As a Gluten Free person you need to change how you approach the social aspect of food.

There is so much to be said about this topic. Think about every social gathering you have ever attended. There was food there, right? Guess what? As a Gluten Free person you will have to be very cautious about what you eat at these social gatherings. Also be prepared not to eat anything at some of these events. Whenever you have the opportunity, when eating out with friends or family, offer up restaurants that you know have good Gluten Free options. When you don't have the option to choose the restaurant, do some quick research online to figure out what will be safe.

12. Be prepared that not everyone will get it right away.

When you decide to live a Gluten Free lifestyle know that not everyone will understand. Some friends may think you are just on a fad diet to lose weight, your aunt may think you are strange because you don't eat her biscuits and your friends may find it odd that you ask so many questions at restaurants. If eating Gluten Free makes you feel better and improves your health, than that is all the evidence you need. Do what you can to educate those around you about why you are living Gluten Free. Help them to understand how sick you were before, but know that there may just be people that don't get it. That is fine. I would just caution you to not eat at their house!

13. You aren't on a fad diet; you are taking care of your body.

Living a Gluten Free lifestyle isn't about shedding some pounds. If living Gluten Free makes you feel better, then do it. For people with Celiac Disease or Gluten allergies the consequences of eating Gluten can put you in the hospital, make you very ill, lead to osteoporosis or even cancer. Find out more at www.Celiac.org.

14. Don't lick envelopes.

Oddly enough wheat is used in many types of glue, including the glue on envelopes. Some envelope glue is made from a natural source called glue Arabic, while others are made with starches like wheat, rice and corn. If you look at a box of envelopes there is no ingredient list, so there is no way to tell if those envelopes have wheat in the glue. To be safe use tape, have someone else lick your envelopes or use a wet paper towel to seal envelopes.

15. Be prepared for your tastes to change once you go Gluten Free.

Once you start eating Gluten Free foods, you will be surprised how your food preferences change. You will start to enjoy foods you wouldn't even eat before. It seems that as you close the door to Gluten, you open doors to new foods. I have a list of foods I never ate in my Gluten eating days that are now part of my regular diet. Be brave and try new things. You may find out you enjoy them.

16. The longer you are Gluten Free the stronger your body will react when it does ingest Gluten.

Living a Gluten Free lifestyle is all or nothing, especially if the life choice is based on a health reason. The longer you go without Gluten the better you allow your body to heal. For some people it can take years for their body to recover from the damage caused by Gluten, for others some of the damage cannot be undone. All of this means that if you cheat or get Glutened further into your Gluten Free journey, expect the reaction to be stronger than you are used to. After years of being Gluten Free it will take me days to get over a Gluten exposure.

17. Don't share a drink with a Gluten-eater.

Do not drink after someone who has been eating Gluten. Like it or not, backwash does happen and little pieces of Gluten could be floating around in the glass. Little kids are the worst at this! In our house my drinks are never shared with little, messy mouths. If you are out and a Gluten-friend orders a fun drink and wants you to try it, the safest option is to politely decline. Order your own drink and enjoy it, knowing it is safe.

18. Play-doh® has Gluten in it.

This favorite toy of children around the world is made from flour, water, salt, boric acid and mineral oil. Depending on how sensitive you are to Gluten, you may just want to avoid this modeling compound and buy something else. You can even find recipes to make your own

Gluten Free Play-doh®. If you do come in contact with the colorful stuff, make sure to thoroughly wash your hands and under your finger nails. Also wipe down any surfaces that came in contact with the Play-doh®.

19. Find a support group to help you.

Living a Gluten Free lifestyle can be hard. You will need support from people who are living this life. You can attend local support groups or find support online. It is so valuable to have people who understand what it feels like to walk into a birthday party and have to pass on the cake or avoid pizza at the work luncheon. It is also helpful to have people to share recommendations about products and restaurants. Connect with other parents who are feeding their children Gluten Free to get advice on how to deal with schools and teachers. You do not want to walk this journey alone.

20. Attend Gluten Free expos and events.

For a small price, you can spend hours walking around an expo where you can eat everything! Imagine not having to ask, "Is that Gluten Free?" It is so freeing to be able eat whatever you see. Aside from the freedom to eat, you will also get to try so many products, and decide what you like and don't like. This will save you so much money. Another benefit is the load of samples and coupons you will take away. You will easily get your money back just in the free samples you eat and take home. If you are within driving distance of a Gluten Free event or expo it is worth the trip.

21. Use Gluten Free lipstick, lip gloss, and chap stick.

What you put on your lips, you ingest. This means if you use lip cosmetics that have Gluten in them, you are ingesting Gluten and making yourself sick. Make sure to read the labels on your cosmetics and toss any with Gluten in them. Also, actively seek cosmetics that are Gluten Free. There are some really good products out there that do not fill your body with Gluten and other junk.

22. Menu planning helps save you time and stress when eating Gluten Free.

Creating a weekly menu plan will save you time, stress, and money. This will allow you to know you have a plan, grocery shop to this plan, and know what food you have in the house to eat. When life gets crazy you can move meals around as needed. The good news is you have options and all the ingredients you need to make those meals.

23. Make sure your vitamins and medicines are Gluten Free.

Gluten ingredients are cheap fillers and help make things stick. Notify your doctor and pharmacist that you are Gluten Free. This will help them better prescribe you safe medicine. This also applies to over-the-counter medicines, so make sure you read the label and do your research. When in doubt contact the company and find out what is safe for you to take.

24. Going Gluten Free doesn't mean you will lose weight.

Living a Gluten Free lifestyle does not guarantee weight loss. For many people, it means they get to finally gain weight because their body is now able to absorb the nutrients in food. If you are looking for an easy way to drop a few pounds, going Gluten Free isn't a guaranteed fix. Living Gluten Free is about making better choices for your body and to allowing it to heal from the damage Gluten has caused.

25. Add more protein, fiber, calcium, and vegetables to your diet.

When you remove Gluten, you need to make sure you add good things back into your diet. Seek out naturally Gluten Free products to increase in your diet. This means things like meat, fiber, calcium and vegetables.

26. Just because something is Gluten Free, doesn't mean it is necessarily healthy.

When a packaged product is labeled Gluten Free, that does means it is safe for you to eat, it doesn't necessarily mean it is good for you. Gluten Free cookies still have calories. Gluten Free bread is also higher in calories than regular bread. All things in moderation, no matter what your lifestyle may be.

27. Be prepared for the Gluten-eating dreams.

Do you dream of Gluten? This may be the oddest part of going Gluten Free, in my opinion. During the day you diligently work to plan your meals and snacks to make sure you have safe food options, but wait until you go to bed! One random night you may dream about eating a big pizza or fried chicken or whatever Gluten item your mind comes up with; this will freak you out. There have been many mornings where I wake up frantic because I can't figure out if the dream was real and if I had really just eaten Gluten. When this happens send me a tweet (@ImaCeliac), so we can laugh about it together.

In the Kitchen

28. Buy squeeze condiments to avoid cross-contamination.

   Cross-contamination is a huge issue for people living Gluten Free. If you use a knife to get butter out of the same container your son buttered his regular bread with, you can make yourself sick. To be safe, try to buy as many squeeze condiments as possible. Try and avoid any jar condiments and if you do buy them, clearly label which ones are Gluten Free. A sharpie marker or colored dot stickers work great for this purpose.

29. Throw away any wooden utensils, cutting boards, and serving dishes.

   Wood is porous and can hold Gluten. If you have wooden items in your kitchen that were used in your Gluten cooking days, you will need to get rid of them. Your trusty wooden spoon that has seen countless batches of Gluten cookies needs to be retired. Again, remember Gluten is sticky and will hang on to these items.

30. If you don't know how to cook, now is a good time to learn.

Eating out Gluten Free is an option, but cooking meals at home is the safest and most economical option when eating Gluten Free. So break out your pots, pans, baking sheets, and slow cooker. It is time to start cooking! There are a ton of great resources available for beginners that range from cookbooks, how-to books and even YouTube videos. Find a friend that is a good cook and have them show you around a few dishes. Community colleges also offer cooking classes to people of all skill levels. Ultimately, preparing your own Gluten Free food is the best way to know it is safe.

31. Gluten Free cooking is made easy with a slow cooker.

Remember that large, oval shaped slow cooker you got for graduation or as a wedding present? This will be a huge help with Gluten Free cooking. Using slow cookers saves you tons of time, energy and money! Before you head out the door in the morning throw in some meat, some veggies, and a sauce in the slow cooker. When you come home after work your house smells great and dinner is ready. We use the slow cooker at least once a week. You can find so many great recipes that utilize the slow cooker.

32. You don't have to throw out your grandma's recipe cards.

Just because you are Gluten Free doesn't mean you can't use the recipes you used to love. You will just need to make some ingredient substitutions. When it comes to baking there are many different Gluten Free flours and flour blends available. You will even use different flours for different recipes. There are also great Gluten Free products available to help you recreate those family favorites. Whether you need cream of chicken soup, soy sauce, breadcrumbs, or pasta, you can find a substitute and make those treasured meals.

33. Put Gluten Free food items on the top shelf in the pantry and fridge.

To avoid cross-contamination in your house, place Gluten Free items on the top shelves in case of spills or crumbs. You don't want to have to throw away good Gluten Free food because regular soy sauce got on it when the bottle fell over. Or what if the box of Gluten crackers sends crumbs flying all over the shelves below? Goodbye Gluten Free food. It can also be helpful to color code or label Gluten Free items so everyone in the family knows it is safe.

34. Wash your counter tops after Gluten has been on them.

Gluten likes to fly around in little particles and stick to whatever it can find. This means that you need to wipe everything in your kitchen down before you prepare a Gluten

Free meal. Alcohol or bleach is best to use on surfaces in your kitchen since Gluten is sticky and stubborn. Keep a spray bottle or wipes out so clean up is easy.

35. Don't share a toaster with Gluten-filled bread.

When you go Gluten Free it is time to buy a new toaster. You can keep the old one for the Gluten eaters in the house but you need a dedicated toaster just for Gluten Free products. And remember most Gluten Free bread products hold up better if they are toasted first. A double-layered toaster oven can be an option as long as it is clearly labeled that only Gluten Free food goes on the top shelf. Even Gluten crumbs can make you sick.

36. Label condiments so people know what is Gluten Free and what is not.

The labels can be fancy with cool Gluten Free stickers or as simple as a permanent marker.   However you approach this task, just make sure it is clear what is Gluten Free and what is regular. If someone sticks a knife in the Gluten Free mayonnaise, spreads it on regular bread, then hits the jar for more mayonnaise with the same knife, the jar is no longer Gluten Free.

37. Use a separate colander for Gluten Free pasta.

To help avoid cross-contamination, have a colander for regular Gluten pasta and one for Gluten Free pasta. This will keep you safe from the random piece of spaghetti that is stuck in one of the holes. If you have to use the same colander, make sure you drain the Gluten Free pasta before the Gluten pasta and that you thoroughly clean it after each use.

38. Don't lick your fingers; you don't know what you may have just touched.

If Gluten is in your world, don't lick your fingers. You don't know if the surface you just touched is clean. For example the refrigerator handle may have Gluten on it if someone in your house touched it after eating Gluten. Check Wikipedia on this one if you don't believe me.

39. Make everyone wash their hands before getting ice out of the ice maker.

No one in the house needs to grab for some ice without first washing their hands. Remember that Gluten is sticky and will hang onto fingers and then fall into an ice bin. You can also buy an ice scoop to avoid this Gluten cross-contamination issue. If you have an ice dispenser on the front of the fridge this will also help. It may also be helpful to put a post-it note on the ice bin for family and friends with a reminder to wash their hands.

40. Give quinoa a chance.

Quinoa is very popular right now as a superfood. Quinoa is a grain full of protein, dietary fiber, iron and magnesium. It is naturally Gluten Free and great for you. It is a great alternative to rice or pasta. You can mix it in with vegetables, meat and a number of sauces. Quinoa is very easy to make and tastes great. It is very versatile and will easily take on the flavors you add to it. Search the Internet for great recipes on how to use this powerful grain.

41. One key item for Gluten Free baking is parchment paper.

Parchment paper is a huge help when baking Gluten Free. You can use any old metal baking sheet, cover it with parchment paper and you are good to go. Parchment paper is also super helpful to avoid having your baked goods stick to pans. You can also invest in the silicone baking mats if you prefer.

Gluten Free Shopping

42. Shop the perimeter of the grocery store.

This is a commonly used saying to help you know where to typically find food items that are naturally Gluten Free. If you walk the perimeter of most grocery stores you will find fruit, vegetables, meats, and dairy products. When you first go Gluten Free these items will be your staples. There are plenty of good Gluten Free food items that you can find down the isles like quinoa, rice, and sauces. But the place to start is with your basic fruit, veggies, meats, and dairy.

43. Regular oats are often cross-contaminated.

When people with Celiac Disease first go Gluten Free it is recommended that they hold off on eating oats for a while. This helps their body heal. When you are ready to eat oats, only use oat products labeled Gluten Free. Most all rolled oats or quick cooking oats have been cross-contaminated with flour. Be sure to check any granola products as well to ensure they use Gluten Free oats.

44. Gluten likes to hide in food.

Gluten likes to hide in tricky places and food manufacturers use it because it is cheap filler and helps to hold ingredients together. Food labels only have to identify the top 8 allergens, so Gluten in its non-wheat forms is not labeled. (At the time this book was written Gluten Free labeling was in the works but nothing was finalized.) Here is a list of ingredients and foods to watch for: soy sauce, salad dressings, marinades, caramel color, natural flavorings, spelt, lunchmeat, cereal, candy, and licorice. If you are concerned about an ingredient in a food it is best to contact the manufacturer to find out what is in the food.

45. Gluten Free packaged food is expensive.

Expect sticker shock when you go Gluten Free grocery shopping for packaged foods. The bread is half the size of a regular Gluten loaf and twice the price. The pasta is $3.00 a box instead of $1.00 for regular Gluten pasta. The list continues, so be prepared to have to pay more. It is essential to read reviews about products to know what is worth buying. You don't want to buy a $7 box of cookies to find out they taste like cardboard.

46. Try different Gluten Free pasta brands.

There are a number of great Gluten Free pastas available. The pastas can be corn, rice, quinoa, flaxseed, or millet based. Try different brands and different blends to see what works best for you. I find that if you plan to bake the pasta it is best to use multi-grain pastas as they hold up better to the longer cooking times. When boiling the Gluten Free pasta, it helps to add some vegetable or olive oil to the water to keep the pasta from not sticking. Also, rinse the pasta well for best success before adding sauce.

47. Find a Gluten Free cup-for-cup flour mix you like.

Shop around and try different Gluten Free all-purpose flour blends to see which ones work the best for your recipes. Some blends are rice based, others potato, others cassava and others bean flour based. Find a blend that works for you and stick with it. To save money you can also create your own Gluten Free flour blend. When using Gluten Free flours don't neglect xanthum gum or another gum to help your baked goods stick together and rise.

48. Some blended teas have Gluten in them so do your research.

Oddly enough some teas have Gluten in them. Like anything you put in or on your body, read the label. Make sure the teas you drink are safe for you. Try to avoid teas with too many additives and stick with natural teas.

49. Gluten Free bread is found in the freezer section of the grocery store.

If you are looking to buy Gluten Free bread products, head to the freezer section of your local health food or grocery store. There are a number of great brands to choose from, but 98% of them reside in the freezer section. This also means when you take the bread home you want to keep it in the freezer until you are ready to use it. Gluten Free bread also does best if you lightly toast it before you eat it. If you do leave Gluten Free bread products out, the shelf life is about three days.

Eating out Gluten Free

50. Whenever you are invited to an event with food, offer to bring a dish.

When you are invited over to a friend's house for dinner, they will want to make you something that you can eat. They will be very well meaning in their intentions to prepare a tasty Gluten Free meal for you. However, the chances of cross-contamination being present are very high. Offer to bring a dish or two to the meal; this will make sure there is at least one thing you will be able to eat. Desserts are very often the hardest things to make Gluten Free due to flour being used in most baked desserts. I will often bring a side dish and a dessert to a friend's house. I have found this helps alleviate some of the stress for the host as well.

51. Don't eat anything that had Gluten scraped off of it.

If you view Gluten as rat poison it helps you better visualize how to avoid it. For example, if someone hands you a salad with regular croutons on it and suggests you take them off, it will be easier to visualize how this is a bad idea. Maybe you are given a sandwich with a bun and told to take the bread off and just to eat the insides. If food is wrapped in rat poison or had rat poison on top if it, you wouldn't eat it, right? The same applies to Gluten and food. Once Gluten has come into contact with food, no amount of scraping can guarantee it is safe.

52. If you are paying for a meal you are entitled to a safe Gluten Free meal.

If you having a catered meal, there is no reason why it cannot be Gluten Free. It only takes a quick phone call or email to notify the establishment that you need a Gluten Free meal. You may end up paying $30 for a plate of grilled vegetables, but at least you get to eat something safe. It is also important when you arrive to notify the catering staff that you need a Gluten Free meal and let then know where you are sitting.

53. It is possible to eat out at a restaurant and eat Gluten Free.

You can eat at certain restaurants and enjoy a safe, Gluten Free meal. However, this takes some work on your part. You need to do your research online to see what your

Gluten Free options are and what you need to tell the manager. Read reviews online and use Gluten Free apps to help you find restaurants that do Gluten Free well. Try to avoid walking into a restaurant blind. If you do, be prepared to eat a plain salad and baked potato.

54. Think outside the bun.

Gluten Free bread isn't always readily available. So when it comes sandwich or burger time, think outside the bun. Some creative alternatives include lettuce leaves, Gluten Free corn tortillas, Gluten Free waffles, or kale leaves. Try to find other ways to enjoy the goodness inside the sandwich without the bread.

55. Have a list of safe restaurants where you can eat.

Having a list of restaurants you have eaten at successfully is key to eating out Gluten Free. Make sure your list includes both fast food chains and sit down restaurants. This list is a huge help when you are traveling as well. If you find a chain of restaurants that do Gluten Free well, have it as a fall back no matter what city you are in.

56. You can still get Glutened at restaurants you trust.

It is sad but true that even in a restaurant with a Gluten Free prep area, a Gluten Free menu and well-trained staff you can still get Glutened. Eating out does come with a risk. You can't guarantee everything is 100% safe and prepared properly unless you are in a 100% Gluten Free restaurant (of which I only know of five nationwide). Do the best you can to ask questions when you order, help educate the staff of your needs and then just cross your fingers. If you do get sick or detect Gluten in your meal, the manager needs to know about it. At one Italian restaurant chain, I found a regular spaghetti noodle mixed in my Gluten Free penne noodles. I immediately stopped eating and let the manager know. They apologized and didn't charge me for the meal. However, at this point the damage was done. My point is, you can eat out at restaurants and eat Gluten Free but even with the best of intentions sometimes things can still go wrong.

57. If French fries are fried in a shared fryer with breaded items they are not Gluten Free fries.

The bad news is most restaurants only have one large fryer that has shared oil. What this means for you is that if someone's flour, breaded chicken tenders were cooked in that oil, the French fries are not Gluten Free. Remember Gluten is sticky and will remain in the oil and can attach to your fries. The fries themselves may have no Gluten ingredients to them, but once they hit the shared fryer they are cross-contaminated. So only eat Gluten Free fried foods that are cooked in a dedicated allergen fryer. You will be surprised that there are some restaurants that can accommodate you.

58. At restaurants ask to speak to the manager about safe Gluten Free options.

When eating out your chances of enjoying a safe Gluten Free meal will be higher if you can talk directly to a manager. The managers are better aware of the kitchen prep methods and ingredients than the average server. It is also helpful to use the word "allergy" rather than

Celiac Disease or Gluten Sensitivity. People understand the severity of allergies so it can be powerful to tell the manager you have a Gluten Allergy. Ask lots of questions, find out how food is prepared, ask about the fryers, and ask about the marinades. Work together to find the best meal for you to enjoy.

59. When eating with crowds, where multiple dishes are on a table, get your plate first.

If you are at a large food gathering, try to cut to the front of the line and fill your plate first. This will make sure the serving spoons are not mixed between dishes. Make sure you fill your plate up with all you plan to eat, as a second trip to the food table would be dangerous. Make sure you ask questions to know which dishes on the table are safe for you to eat.

Gluten Free Travel Tips

60. Take safe Gluten Free food with you wherever you go.

Never leave home without taking Gluten Free food with you. This can be a snack bar, travel mix, or your favorite Gluten Free treats. Keep a stash of food in your car, your office, your purse, and wherever you travel. As a Gluten Free person you do not always know where you will find safe food, so it is best to carry some with you.

61. Use phone apps to tell you where to eat and what is Gluten Free at different restaurants.

Aside from having a list of Gluten Free restaurants you know are safe, phone apps can also help you find safe places to eat. Smart phones are a huge resource for helping you find safe, Gluten Free products, and restaurants that have Gluten Free menus. You can use Google to find quick options or use many downloadable apps. Some apps I use include: Find Me Gluten Free, Yelp, UrbanSpoon, iCanEat, and YoDish.

62. Don't eat the snacks on planes; even the peanuts have a wheat allergy warning.

When you are traveling keep safe food with you. Most of the foods on airplanes have Gluten ingredients or wheat allergy warnings. It is best not to rely on the airline for your inflight snack. If you are going on a long flight that includes a meal, make sure you notify the airline of your Gluten Free needs in advance. It is also best to bring enough snacks with you in case the meal is not safe.

63. Plan ahead when traveling.

Do your research before you travel. Find out what grocery stores are close by where you can restock your Gluten Free resources. Ask the hotel for a room with a mini-fridge and microwave so you can prepare a safe Gluten Free breakfast. Also find out what restaurants are available in the area with Gluten Free menus. A loaf of Gluten Free bread, peanut butter, some fruit, hummus, and some snack bars can get you through a trip. You may end up traveling with more food than clothes!

Succeed at Living Gluten Free

Final Tips

64. Focus on what you can eat, not on what you can't eat.

Stay positive about living Gluten Free. If you focus on all the foods you can't eat, life will be very depressing. Focus on all the naturally tasty Gluten Free foods you get to enjoy. Find Gluten Free bakeries and restaurants that make amazing treats. Enjoy the new community of friends you have made that understand your new lifestyle. Seek out new adventures that incorporate your lifestyle. You can live Gluten Free and enjoy your life.

65. Wash your hands and read labels.

Two of the keys to living Gluten Free are to always wash your hands before you eat and read the labels of the products you eat. You never know what may be lurking on the surface you just touched, so be safe and wash your hands or use an alcohol based hand gel before you eat. Make reading food labels your new hobby. Get good at being able to quickly scan for Gluten ingredients. If you know what you are putting in your mouth, you will be able to enjoy your food safely.

Wrapping it up

My hope is that these 65 tips have given you insight into how to Succeed at Living Gluten Free. It is possible to live a fulfilling life without Gluten. You will be able to enjoy very good food. You will be able to travel the world and still eat Gluten Free. Don't let living Gluten Free drag you down, be empowered by this new lifestyle and how good you feel because of it.

You are not alone.
You can do this!

Pam Jordan's Bio

Pam Jordan was diagnosed with Celiac Disease in January 2011 after struggling for fifteen years with symptoms. Her journey included diagnosis of Irritable Bowl Syndrome, Depression and Infertility. Finally after getting tested for Celiac Disease she was given the answer to all her health problems. There was no cure but there was treatment, a Gluten Free Lifestyle. Within two weeks of going Gluten Free Pam was a new person.

Pam has a passion for living Gluten Free and wants to help others on their journey. On her blog, ImaCeliac.com, she writes weekly menus, creates recipes, writes product reviews, recipe reviews, travel tips and hosts giveaways.

Pam is a financial executive with an MBA by day and a wife and mom by night. She enjoys spending time with her family, running and helping the Gluten Free community.

Other books by Pam Jordan

Family Approved Gluten Free Recipes
A cookbook with over 50 easy to make
recipes, using simple ingredients that your
whole family will love. These recipes
have easy to follow directions and taste
great!

You can purchase Pam's cookbook on
Amazon.

It's Celiac Disease, Now What?
Is an eBook for the newly diagnosed
Celiac. It goes in-depth about how to
clean your kitchen, how to grocery shop,
how to eat out and answers many more of
your questions.

You can purchase this eBook on Pam's
website, Imaceliac.com.

Gluten Free One Dish Meals
Is an eBook with a week's worth of dinners that can be prepared in one pot, one skillet, one casserole dish, or one slow cooker. These recipes are big crowd pleasers.

You can purchase this eBook on Pam's website, Imaceliac.com.

Contact Pam Jordan
www.ImaCeliac.com
www.Twitter.com/Imaceliac
www.Facebook.com/Imaceliac

Gluten Free Resources

Celiac Disease Foundation
www.Celiac.org

National Foundation of Celiac Awareness
www.CeliacCentral.org

Gluten Intolerance Groups
www.gluten.net

Celiac Spruce Association
www.csaceliacs.info

Create your own tips to Succeed at Living Gluten Free!